Cambridge Elements ≡

Elements of Improving Quality and Safety in Healthcare
edited by
Mary Dixon-Woods,* Katrina Brown,* Sonja Marjanovic,†
Tom Ling,† Ellen Perry,* and Graham Martin*
*THIS Institute (The Healthcare Improvement Studies Institute)
†RAND Europe

SIMULATION
AS AN IMPROVEMENT
TECHNIQUE

Victoria Brazil,[1,2] Eve Purdy,[1,2]
and Komal Bajaj[3]

[1] Translational Simulation Collaborative, Faculty of Health Sciences and
Medicine, Bond University
[2] Emergency Department, Gold Coast University Hospital
[3] NYC Health + Hospitals

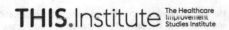
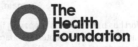

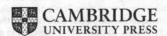

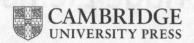

Shaftesbury Road, Cambridge CB2 8EA, United Kingdom

One Liberty Plaza, 20th Floor, New York, NY 10006, USA

477 Williamstown Road, Port Melbourne, VIC 3207, Australia

314–321, 3rd Floor, Plot 3, Splendor Forum, Jasola District Centre,
New Delhi – 110025, India

103 Penang Road, #05–06/07, Visioncrest Commercial, Singapore 238467

Cambridge University Press is part of Cambridge University Press & Assessment,
a department of the University of Cambridge.

We share the University's mission to contribute to society through the pursuit of
education, learning and research at the highest international levels of excellence.

www.cambridge.org
Information on this title: www.cambridge.org/9781009338165

DOI: 10.1017/9781009338172

First published 2023

A catalogue record for this publication is available from the British Library.

ISBN 978-1-009-33816-5 Paperback
ISSN 2754-2912 (online)
ISSN 2754-2904 (print)

Cambridge University Press & Assessment has no responsibility for the persistence
or accuracy of URLs for external or third-party internet websites referred to in this
publication and does not guarantee that any content on such websites is, or will
remain, accurate or appropriate.

Every effort has been made in preparing this Element to provide accurate and up-to-date information
that is in accord with accepted standards and practice at the time of publication. Although case
histories are drawn from actual cases, every effort has been made to disguise the identities of the
individuals involved. Nevertheless, the authors, editors, and publishers can make no warranties that
the information contained herein is totally free from error, not least because clinical standards are
constantly changing through research and regulation. The authors, editors, and publishers therefore
disclaim all liability for direct or consequential damages resulting from the use of material contained in
this Element. Readers are strongly advised to pay careful attention to information provided by the
manufacturer of any drugs or equipment that they plan to use.

Simulation as an Improvement Technique

Elements of Improving Quality and Safety in Healthcare

DOI: 10.1017/9781009338172
First published online: January 2023

Victoria Brazil,[1,2] Eve Purdy,[1,2] and Komal Bajaj[3]
[1] Translational Simulation Collaborative, Faculty of Health Sciences and Medicine, Bond University
[2] Emergency Department, Gold Coast University Hospital
[3] NYC Health + Hospitals

Author for correspondence: Victoria Brazil, vbrazil@bond.edu.au

Abstract: Historically simulation was used as an education and training technique in healthcare, but now has an emerging role in improving quality and safety. Simulation-based techniques can be applied to help understand healthcare settings and the practices and behaviours of those who work in them. Simulation-based interventions can help to improve care and outcomes – for example, by improving readiness of teams to respond effectively to situations or to improve skill and speed. Simulation can also help test planned interventions and infrastructural changes, allowing possible vulnerabilities and risks to be identified and addressed. Challenges include cost, resources, training, and evaluation, and the lack of connection between the simulation and improvement fields, both in practice and in scholarship. The business case for simulation as an improvement technique remains to be established. This Element concludes by offering a way forward for simulation in practice and for future scholarly directions to improve the approach. This title is also available as Open Access on Cambridge Core.

Keywords: simulation, translational simulation, healthcare improvement, health professions education, outcomes

ISBNs: 9781009338165 (PB), 9781009338172 (OC)
ISSNs: 2754-2912 (online), 2754-2904 (print)

Contents

1 Introduction

Simulation has been employed as an educational technique in healthcare, but is rapidly evolving as an approach for healthcare improvement. This Element reviews its current and potential future use. We outline the origins of simulation as an educational technique and characterise the increasing interest in, and use of, simulation as a way of improving care. We show how simulation can be used to explore working environments, and the practices and behaviours of those who work in them, to improve clinical performance and outcomes, to test planned interventions and infrastructural changes, and to help professionals learn about, and embed a culture of, improvement. We discuss the challenges of using simulation as an improvement technique, including the current lack of connection between the simulation and healthcare improvement fields – both in practice and in scholarship. We conclude by offering a way forward for simulation as an improvement technique in practice and for future scholarly directions to improve the method.

2 Healthcare Simulation as an Improvement Technique

This section provides an explanation of terminology, methods, and the scope of the term 'simulation'. We consider the history of simulation in healthcare – and its traditional role as an education and training technique focused on patient safety. Building on these traditions, simulation is now emerging as a method for examining and improving systems. Few published real-world examples have been described or evaluated in sufficient depth to be considered exemplars, so we offer in-depth, hypothetical case vignettes to provide granular illustration of the method and the diverse techniques employed under the umbrella term of simulation. We give an overview of efforts by the community of practice in healthcare simulation to crystallise these approaches into a consistent method and to explore the relationship with existing healthcare improvement methods, including addressing relationships, reliability, and risk.

2.1 Definition and Description of Healthcare Simulation

Simulation as an imitation of a situation or process has a long history within fields such as aviation and construction. Since the turn of the century, simulation has been adopted in healthcare as 'a technique that creates a situation or environment to allow persons to experience a representation of a real event for the purpose of practice, learning, evaluation, testing, or to gain understanding of systems or human actions'.[1]

In his seminal work, *The future vision of simulation in health care*,[2] Gaba outlines 11 dimensions that highlight the various applications of simulation.

Positing that 'simulation is a technique, not a technology', Gaba underscores the diversity of simulation techniques. Simulation can look like many different things, in different places, with different people. In a medical school, for example, students use simulation when they practise suturing on task trainers – plastic models with fake skin. Within a hospital context, a simulation may be conducted 'in situ' (within a real clinical space) with a manikin acting as the patient. Equipped with technology to emulate a heartbeat, vital signs, realistic lungs, and electronic haptic (touch) feedback, this could allow an interventional cardiology team to catheterize the heart while the intensive care team resuscitates the patient. In a resuscitation bay, an emergency department team standing around an empty stretcher could be engaging in a brief mental simulation exercise to start their shift.

In short, there is no single recipe for a simulation programme or simulation exercise. Box 1 describes a hypothetical case vignette of applying simulation to a specific healthcare improvement goal – improving performance in emergencies on a cardiac surgery ward. The vignette illustrates the complexity of the clinical performance being explored and the variety of simulation techniques that might be employed to achieve the improvement goal. In Table 1, we then explore that example through the lens of Gaba's 11 dimensions of simulation.[2]

2.2 How Simulation Became Integrated into Approaches to Improve Quality and Safety

The benefits of healthcare simulation for education and training in a variety of contexts are well described.[4] Historically, simulation was assumed to improve patient safety and care quality through the education of individual healthcare professionals and teams.

Early use of simulation focused on practising procedural skills using part task trainers – for example, using oranges to practise intramuscular injection, plastic arms to practise intravenous cannulation, and plastic head and neck simulators to practise airway management techniques. As technology has improved, educational applications for procedural skills now extend to virtual reality and software-based simulation of complex procedural tasks, such as laparoscopic surgery.

Improving a wider range of clinical skills such as communication is also a common use of simulation. Simulated patients are trained educators acting as patients, recreating everyday and challenging conversations, such as history taking, discussing bad news, or end-of-life conversations, and offering thoughtful feedback to learners in real time.[5]

BOX 1 IMPROVING PERFORMANCE IN EMERGENCIES ON A CARDIAC SURGERY WARD

A cardiac surgery ward wants to improve its ability to respond to a rare but critical event: cardiac arrest in patients after cardiac surgery. This clinical situation requires a functioning ad hoc team, clinical decision-making that falls outside of usual cardiac arrest algorithms, and specific equipment.

Four simulation sessions are organised to take place over the course of a year, with the aim of clinical teams practising together for this critical event, and reflecting on the human factors that contribute to success or failure. A scenario is designed by the simulation delivery team – a group comprised of clinician experts and members with specific simulation technical skills and group facilitation expertise. The scenario outlines stages of the clinical encounter: initial patient deterioration 2 hours after surgery, sudden loss of cardiac output, and recovery after appropriate team interventions.

The simulation delivery team expects that the four sessions will offer a chance for iterative improvement if clinical teams identify opportunities for better teamwork or systems. In each session, staff who would be involved in such a clinical situation are organised to attend the simulation, which is conducted in a bed space in the cardiac surgical ward. Each simulation includes 10 participants from the clinical teams who would come together for this critical event (rapid response registrar and nurse, ward nurses, anaesthetics registrar, intensive care unit registrar, cardiac surgeon, intensive care unit administration clerk, and porterage staff).

Each session involves:

(1) a short pre-briefing for the clinical team, outlining the aims of the exercise and clarifying expectations
(2) the scenario, during which the clinical team is required to recognise the patient deterioration and respond appropriately
(3) a debriefing discussion with the clinical team, facilitated by a member of the simulation delivery team.

The debrief includes addressing any knowledge gaps (educational outcomes) but is mostly focused on supporting the clinical team to identify opportunities for better teamwork, equipment set ups, call systems, and cognitive aids. After each session, the simulation delivery team creates a report on the findings from the simulation and a debrief that is circulated to participants and to departmental leadership.

• In the first simulation, participants identify that having two different cardiac arrest trolleys on the ward leads to confusion.

- In the second simulation, the rapid response registrar voices unfamiliarity with the alterations to the cardiac arrest algorithm for patients after cardiac surgery. This provides the opportunity for the expertise of cardiac surgical ward nurses to be uncovered and amplified in the debrief.
- In the third simulation, a newly designed single cardiac arrest trolley (based on issues identified in the first simulation) is trialled.
- In the final simulation, the facilitator notices that the ward nurse gives the rapid response registrar a cue card when they arrive bedside to remind them of the differences in cardiac arrest management in this particular clinical situation. This card was designed by the ward charge nurse and a rapid response registrar after the second simulation.

Computer-based simulation of patient care scenarios, which require learners to synthesise information and make decisions about investigations and treatments, can improve decision-making and support cognitive aspects of healthcare delivery.[6]

And, in recognition of the critical role of teamwork in healthcare, simulations can be focused on teamwork behaviours. These involve teams of healthcare practitioners caring for a patient to support learning about both common and rare presentations, while providing opportunities to practise role allocation, leadership, and communication within the team.

If appropriately embedded within an educational framework,[7] these examples of simulation-based education can lead to faster and more effective learning without the attendant risks of subjecting patients to practitioners' learning curves. Best practice for educationally focused simulation includes integrating simulation into curricula, capturing clinical variation, allowing repetitive practice, and incorporating useful feedback or time for reflection.[8,9] An exponential growth in educational simulation research since 1980 has also led to an increased emphasis on sound educational principles – for example, maintaining psychological safety for participants and increasing emphasis on debriefing and reflective practice.

Box 2 describes a hypothetical case vignette illustrating the need for simulation activities to be supported by educational frameworks (including assessment) and cultural change to be successful.

Recent years have seen widespread adoption of simulation in healthcare professions' curricula for education, continuing professional development, and team improvement.[9] Here, simulation is seen as an educational adjunct, manifested in a desire for standardised educational opportunities, the need to practise skills before applying them in a clinical environment, and to supplement scarce

Table 1 Applying Gaba's 11 dimensions of simulation[2] to the case vignette in Box 1

Simulation dimension	Description	Example (application of 11 dimensions to the case vignette)
Aims and purposes of the simulation activity	Simulation can be used for education and training, assessment of performance, investigation into organisational practices, investigation of human factors, and institutional change.	To train ward and rapid response teams and to reflect upon the human factors associated with their response to cardiac arrest in patients after cardiac surgery.
Unit of participation	Simulation can be deployed at the individual, team, work unit, or organisational level.	Activity is at the organisational level across several teams, including the ward, intensive care unit, anaesthesia, and cardiac surgery teams.
Experience level of participants	All levels of training from undergraduates to practising healthcare professionals can use simulation.	Participants are practising healthcare professionals.
Healthcare domain	All health specialties, including non-clinical areas, can apply simulation.	Cardiac surgery, intensive care unit, anaesthetics, risk management, environmental services, pastoral care.
Professional discipline of participants	Simulation can be applied to all disciplines within healthcare and is often interprofessional.	Interprofessional
Type of knowledge, skills, attitudes, or behaviours addressed	Conceptual understanding, technical and decision-making skills, or attitudes and	Conceptual understanding of how postoperative cardiac arrest differs from regular cardiac arrest on the wards.

Table 1 (cont.)

Simulation dimension	Description	Example (application of 11 dimensions to the case vignette)
	behaviours can be addressed using simulation.	Explore decision to reopen the chest in the cardiac arrest. Trust between team members. Communication between rapidly constructed team.
The simulated patient's age	Simulation is applicable to every type and age of patient.	Patients include a 4-year-old with a congenital heart defect and a 65-year-old with coronary artery disease.
Technology applicable or required	Simulation can be accomplished through low-technology methods, such as standardised patients (actors), or high-technology options, such as computer-based or full-body electronic simulators.	Manikin-based simulation with cardiorespiratory monitoring and voice. Physical adjustment to the manikin to allow for surgical reopening of the chest, and a fake, beating heart to allow internal cardiac compressions.
Site of simulation	Simulation may take place at home/office through screen-based simulations, in a replica clinical environment such as a simulation centre, or within an actual working unit.	Cardiac surgery ward.

Table 1 (cont.)

Simulation dimension	Description	Example (application of 11 dimensions to the case vignette)
Extent of direct participation	Simulations may be view-only, involve remote-viewing with some level of verbal or haptic interaction, or immersive in nature.	10 participants are directly involved.
Method of feedback used	The opportunity to reflect on a simulated experience greatly increases the impact of the intervention. This can be accomplished through automated critique provided by simulator and by coaching/debriefing during or after the event.	Structured debriefing with an experienced facilitator using an established framework (PEARLS for systems integration)[3] for a large group. Opportunity for additional one-to-one coaching for participants who identify personal learning gaps.

clinical training sites. The educational focus mostly reflects a person-centred approach to safety, in which the purpose of training is to decrease the number of errors by individuals and teams.

Coinciding with the integration of simulation into education has been a growing understanding of the contribution of behaviour and other non-technical skills to team performance in complex health systems.[10–13] Team-based, crew-resource management training that includes simulation has been associated with improved teamwork and confidence among a variety of healthcare teams.[14,15] Such an approach has undoubted value: training for teamwork, communication, and procedural skills is necessary for improved patient care. But there remains limited understanding of how long these improvements persist and what impact they have on clinical outcomes. Further, on their own, educational uses of simulation are unlikely to be sufficient to address the need for more systems-based approaches that are now recognised as fundamental to securing quality and safety.[16]

BOX 2 ATTEMPT TO IMPROVE OPERATING THEATRE EFFICIENCY THROUGH SIMULATION

A hospital wants to improve its operating theatre efficiency. One factor affecting current performance is the time taken for trainees to perform operations, including laparoscopic appendicectomies. Relatively junior trainee surgeons are allowed to perform these procedures, taking on the role of the primary operator, but they may be slow since they are going through a learning curve.

A training programme is developed to improve the skills of trainees through laparoscopic simulation, using both simple task trainers (which trainees can even take home) and highly complex, virtual reality simulators (Figure 1). Attendance at training is variable, due to competing clinical demands on trainee surgeons' time. Trainees who do attend demonstrate rapid improvement in skills. The supervising consultants are aware of the training, but they still consider the laparoscopic appendicectomies on real patients as excellent opportunities for the trainees to practise, and they allow the slow operations to continue. There is no accepted credentialing process to become a primary operator at the institution. Nurses and technical specialist staff in the operating theatre are not involved in any of the training exercises, and administrative staff are not engaged to review the scheduling of operations. After 12 months, no change is demonstrated in operating theatre efficiency.

Those with oversight of the training programme reflect that the lack of robust assessment and credentialing process, and their inability to change supervision practice and operating theatre culture, has meant that the simulation training has had minimal impact on operating theatre efficiency.

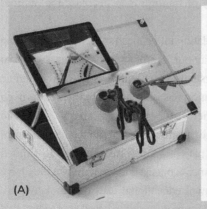 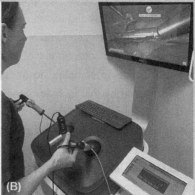

Figure 1 A simple task trainer (A) and a virtual reality simulator (B) for laparoscopic simulation

© *Victoria Brazil*

There is a growing understanding of the positive roles that simulation can play, beyond education and training, in improving quality and safety in organisations. Consistent with Gaba's proposal that 'using simulation to improve safety will require full integration of its applications into the routine structures and practices of health care',[2] there is evidence of increased use of simulation for the express purpose of healthcare improvement, such as identifying latent safety threats or improving processes. The term translational simulation was coined in 2017 to describe those simulation activities 'connected directly with health service priorities and patient outcomes, through interventional, testing and diagnostic functions'.[17] A brief PubMed search shows that in the year 2000, there were 21 publications related to 'simulation and "patient safety"'; in 2021, that same search yielded 741 results. Many institutions, teams, and researchers are realising, honing, and advancing Gaba's original vision.

These shifts are occurring alongside – and to some extent inspired by– the evolution of paradigms for safety thinking. In 2013, a white paper by Hollnagel et al.[18] prompted a shift towards what the authors call a 'Safety II' perspective. They argue that we should cease to focus exclusively on how to stop things going wrong, and emphasise instead why things go right. A Safety I approach to healthcare presumes that things go wrong because of identifiable failures of specific components of a system, but such an approach does not address the contribution of the system as a whole, including its culture and variability.[10–13] By contrast, Safety II focuses on proactively fostering a system that allows as many things as possible to go right, with an effort to continuously anticipate issues and embrace humans as contributors to flexibility and resilience.[10–13] Simulation has emerged over the past decade as having potential to purposefully uphold and complement a Safety II approach.[19–22] This is recognised in the Society for Simulation Healthcare's accreditation of programmes that undertake 'systems integration' simulation:

A category of simulation program accreditation that recognizes programs that demonstrate consistent, planned, collaborative, integrated, and iterative application of simulation-based assessment, research, and teaching activities with systems engineering and risk management principles to achieve excellent bedside clinical care, enhanced patient safety, and improved outcome metrics across the health care system(s).[1]

Many simulation researchers and practitioners embraced this change in the safety paradigm, and began to reconceptualise the role of simulation as going beyond an educational adjunct. Simulation techniques emerged that were system focused[23] and more integrated into improvement approaches.

3 Simulation in Action

This section considers the mechanisms by which simulation can be applied to improving healthcare. As an emerging methodology, there is no consensus on best practice. Expert guidance has been offered on theoretical and practical approaches.[24–29] Recent publications offer operational frameworks and practical toolkits for practitioners of translational simulation.[23,30]

We look at four areas in turn.

- Simulation can be used to *explore working environments* (or the practices and behaviours of those in them) to identify latent safety threats or other opportunities for improvement.
- It may be employed as an *intervention to improve healthcare* through targeted activities focused on clinical performance or outcomes (e.g. time-based targets, resuscitation outcomes, teamwork, culture change, and healthcare professional relationships).
- Simulation may be used as a *technique for testing* planned interventions and changes to infrastructure (e.g. checklists, care pathways, electronic health records, and commissioning new facilities).
- Simulation-based *educational activities* may support healthcare professionals' learning about improvement principles and practice.

3.1 Exploring Working Environments and the Practices and Behaviours of Those in Them

Simulation offers a broad range of opportunities and methods for examining current healthcare practice, including the various factors that shape performance at an individual, team, technology, working environment, or system level.[31,32]

Simulation is an attractive option when study in an actual clinical setting would be difficult due to practical constraints or ethical concerns – for example, interrupting nurses during medication rounds to determine error rates. Increasingly, simulated explorations are now frequently undertaken as part of an initial or ongoing improvement strategy too. Diverse techniques can be employed: for example, task trainers to study procedural skill performance (e.g. a plastic arm that allows for intravenous cannula insertion); scenario-based immersive simulations to study team performance; role play with simulated patients to review communication; and computer modelling simulation to examine patient flow through an emergency department.

Simulations conducted within the actual care setting (in situ simulation[33]) may be particularly valuable in evaluating system performance and identifying latent conditions that pose threats to patient safety. This more naturalistic approach enables participants to practise within the same physical environment, healthcare team, and care processes that are used in real clinical practice. It recognises that clinical practice happens under conditions of 'considerable complexity, change and surprise',[21] which are difficult to capture in dedicated simulation laboratories.

In situ simulation programmes claim to ' ... accomplish ... the dual goals of identifying and remedying [latent safety threats] as well as providing continuous opportunities to deliberately practice technical and non-technical skills'.[33] Parallel exploration may also occur within team relationships, roles, and culture[20,21,34] – which are equally likely sources of latent safety threats to health service performance or safety. A typical approach might involve a hospital department simulating scenarios that are representative of their patient profile and require a team-based approach to care, located within an actual patient care space. Exercises are generally accompanied by a debriefing session in which the professionals involved reflect on their performance and the opportunities and constraints afforded by the physical space and other resources available. Programmes have been conducted in emergency departments, operating theatres, maternity units, general wards, pre-hospital environments, and primary care contexts.

Importantly, simulations that explore working environments are also an opportunity for learning from success,[22] as they enable tacit expertise and examples of positive deviance can be identified and elaborated[35] (the positive deviance approach is explored in another Element in this series[36]). In situ exercises become an opportunity to 'investigate and optimize human activity based on the connected layers of any setting: the embodied competences of the healthcare professionals, the social and organizational rules that guide their actions, and the material aspects of the setting'.[22] As such, we see alignment with trends in patient safety towards Safety II approaches – reinforcing the role of efficient adaptation and organisational resilience in the face of errors and obstacles arising.[37]

Box 3 outlines a hypothetical case vignette in which in situ simulation is used to explore the working environment, latent safety threats, team function, and positive deviance in caring for paediatric patients with anaphylaxis. It illustrates some of the challenges in translating to change in practice.

When using simulation to explore working environments, the delivery methods vary greatly. Scenarios may be conducted in actual patient care areas or nearby to facilitate team attendance. Sessions may be unannounced and unexpected, simulating real response processes, or they may be planned and scheduled in advance.[29] Each design decision is likely to require some trade-offs between the feasibility of conducting simulation exercises in a clinical environment and the veracity of the system-probing function.[38]

> ### Box 3 Managing paediatric anaphylaxis in an emergency department
>
> A paediatric emergency department is interested in improving its management of children presenting with life-threatening anaphylaxis. A series of 10 immersive, team-based simulation sessions are delivered to staff who work in the department, conducted in the departmental resuscitation bay. Due to rosters and staffing, each simulation session involves a different mix of team members, and many staff in the department don't get to participate in any of the sessions. In each simulation, the clinical team is notified of a 5-year-old child en route with a life-threatening allergic reaction. The child (represented by a manikin) arrives in the resuscitation bay 5 minutes later, requiring rapid assessment and treatment with intramuscular adrenaline.
>
> Observation of the clinical team's performance by the simulation delivery team and subsequent debriefing conversations reveal a series of issues: difficulty accessing adrenaline in the appropriate concentration due to the location of the drug cupboard, knowledge gaps within the clinical team about dosage and route of administration, and inadequate pre-briefing before the patient arrives via ambulance. However, the simulation also identifies some better practices by some clinical teams during the scenario: the use of appropriate cognitive aids located on the computer in the room, and earlier calls for help to senior staff.
>
> The simulation delivery team records the issues and prepares a report for departmental leadership with suggestions for changes in practice relating to equipment, environment, and teamwork. After 6 months, some of these suggestions have been actioned, but staff turnover and waning enthusiasm have stalled other improvements.

At present, however, there are no design standards nor even a consensus on terminology.[29] Frequently identified practical challenges include those relating to equipment, medication, use of physical space, and call systems.

Using in situ simulation to explore working environments is a potentially attractive approach in healthcare improvement, but is immature in its methods, consistency, and integration with other improvement strategies. Auerbach et al. report, for example, that most paediatric simulation programmes they surveyed used in situ simulation, but also found inadequacies in how latent safety threats were identified, reported, and acted on.[24] A systematic review of studies reporting in situ simulation activities found that 'approaches to design, delivery, and evaluation of the simulations were highly variable across studies', and that performance measurement practices were suboptimal.[39]

Colman et al. have developed a more standardised approach to simulation-based testing of clinical systems,[40] providing documentation and evaluation tools to help in identifying inefficiencies and risks to safety. But as yet there is no consensus on the best approach. There is also conflicting evidence about whether improvements to working environments are sustained, with some arguing that it is most likely to be effective if seen as a long-term commitment requiring regular participation that is intrinsic to an ongoing patient safety strategy.[27]

3.2 Improving Clinical Performance and Outcomes

Simulation can be applied to a broad range of healthcare targets: anything from a single patient journey at one institution to improvement of system outcomes. The clearest examples include simulation projects designed to improve time-based targets or other easily measurable indicators related to individual patient journeys, such as time to thrombolysis in stroke care,[41] time for trauma patients to go to CT scan,[42] resuscitation outcomes,[43] teamwork in trauma,[44] or success rates in paediatric intubation.[45] Simulations designed for such a purpose may include dedicated educational programmes to improve individual and team performance – for example, deploying part-task training for procedural skills and immersive simulations for team-based tasks, combined with appropriate didactic or other training methods. The hypothetical case vignette in Box 4 is a typical example.

In a review of the clinical outcomes of simulation-based 'mastery learning' (learning that helps students to master or reach a high level of achievement), Griswold-Theodorson et al. identified studies reporting improvements following training interventions, including better performance level, better procedural success rate, reduced patient discomfort, shorter procedure times, reduced error rate, and lower healthcare costs.[46] Reviews of in situ simulation practice have also demonstrated improved patient morbidity and mortality.[47] In situ simulation is likely to be especially important given that outcomes are dependent on how individuals and teams perform within the constraints and opportunities of hospital systems and complex departmental interfaces.

Reported examples of successful improvement programmes often relate to interventions conducted in a single institution, but simulation has the potential to impact healthcare beyond these examples. Simulation may be used to improve healthcare management and policy-making at a state or national level,[48] where the impact is more distributed. Nataraja et al. report a significant national

BOX 4 IMPROVING TIME TO TREATMENT FOR MYOCARDIAL INFARCTION

A multidisciplinary group of health professionals in a regional centre want to improve their 'call-to-balloon' time, which describes the time from receiving a call about a person who is experiencing a myocardial infarction requiring urgent coronary angioplasty and stenting to the person receiving the procedure. Following an audit showing that their local performance was below national benchmarks, a group of pre-hospital providers (e.g. ambulance crews), emergency department staff, and cardiac catheterisation laboratory (cath lab) teams work with simulation experts to design a simulation programme to improve.

Weekly simulations are conducted for 2 months, each involving a simulated call to the ambulance communication centre, prioritisation, dispatch of ambulance crew, and provision of initial treatments. An actor is employed to be the patient with a heart attack. The patient is transported to the emergency department and then transferred to the cath lab. All members of the clinical team are aware that their target time is 60 minutes. The staff members participating in the simulations are drawn from those rostered to work on those days, so each session involves a different team.

Over a period of 2 months, the call-to-balloon times reduce. Teams find better ways to communicate and to process tasks in parallel, such as preparing the emergency department and cath lab after initial pre-hospital reading of the electrocardiogram. Emergency department staff become more familiar with the cath lab environment and can help the clinical team to set up faster before the procedure.

In an evaluation, healthcare staff report that they are more confident, have enjoyed the simulations, and have changed their practice as a result. While this process has improved call-to-balloon median time for real patients by 20% in the 6 months following the simulations, mortality and length of stay at 12 months is unchanged, indicating that there is further work to do. The lack of improvement in patient-centred outcomes may suggest other factors (e.g. catheterization lab procedures, provision of evidence-based critical care, and rehab practices) may be important next targets for improvement.

improvement in the management of paediatric intussusception (an acute bowel emergency) in Myanmar following the introduction of a focused, simulation-based intervention.[49] Preparing a disaster plan or evaluating strategies to minimise infections during a pandemic such as COVID-19 might involve computer modelling techniques, combined with live simulations to test protocols for safe patient care,[25] and training simulations to determine if personal protective equipment is adequate.[50]

Relationships and culture within and between healthcare teams are less frequent targets for simulation-based interventions, despite the recognised role they both play in health system performance. In one study of a relationship-based approach to improve trauma care at an institution, Purdy et al.[34] illustrate the considerable impact of regular interprofessional, multidisciplinary, in situ simulation on the relational aspects of care and the development of a collaborative culture.[20] Another study of a programme involving regular emergency department simulation showed that simulation is a place to foster familiarity and psychological safety, which can have a direct impact on clinicians' work in real clinical settings.[51] For further discussion of some of the issues relating to culture in healthcare, see the Element on making culture change happen.[52]

Overall, the simulation techniques used for targeting system improvements are variable – combinations of in situ simulation, educationally focused simulation in dedicated facilities, procedural skills practice, and scenario-based team training. The design requires clarity on the hopefully meaningful target(s) and appreciation of the relative benefits of various simulation methods to achieve improvement, while being feasible and cost-effective to implement.[17,28] Simulation itself is agnostic towards healthcare improvement frameworks and is frequently one part of a more comprehensive improvement strategy,[45] which is pragmatic and appropriate, but which makes it difficult to ascertain the specific impact of the simulation elements on the overall effectiveness of the approach.[26] Liberati et al. highlight this interrelationship by outlining how a host of quality and safety mechanisms within a maternity unit were 'nurtured and sustained' through the simulation-based Practical Obstetric Multi-Professional Training (PROMPT) programme.[53] The PROMPT course is focused on multi-professional teams learning how to manage obstetric emergencies, working on their own labour ward, using their own emergency equipment, local procedures, and systems.[54]

3.3 Testing Planned Interventions and Infrastructural Changes

Simulation can enable evaluation of the feasibility, safety, acceptability, or effectiveness of planned interventions, new healthcare facilities, and changes to infrastructure. This provides opportunities to develop and test ergonomics and workflows, and to identify human factors flaws and latent safety threats before going live or being introduced into the real clinical environment.[31,40,55–57] Effectively designed simulations can also be used to test new processes. For example, they have been used to test cognitive aids for emergencies,[58] guidelines for massive transfusion and other care pathways, and the introduction of new equipment or bundles, such as boxes for the management of postpartum haemorrhage.[59] Strategies can encompass a range of techniques and targets, with success dependent on the authenticity of the simulation and the adequacy of data collection.[55] Simulation can be used as one part of a mixed-methods design, where data collected through simulation can be triangulated with other sources of information and intelligence.[31]

Testing may include tabletop mock-ups, full-scale recreations of facilities, and individuals or teams working within test environments to varying degrees of realism. This requires more than a single event – it requires a strategy for testing and data collection. Petrosoniak et al.[57] propose a 'design thinking' approach, with multimodal simulation techniques and an emphasis on end user engagement, to iteratively test and improve planned changes to a trauma resuscitation bay in an emergency department. Although frameworks have been described in the literature,[40] there are no endorsed standards and no accepted consensus approach for using simulation to test new healthcare facilities.

However, some important examples are appearing. Prior to the opening of a newly constructed paediatric outpatient clinic, Colman et al.[60] conducted 31 simulated scenarios over 3 months to identify system flaws (latent safety threats) that posed a potential risk to patients. Failure mode and effects analysis was used to prioritise threats. In all, the authors identified 334 latent safety threats, including 36 'very high priority' threats. High-priority examples included emergency preparedness and the emergency notification system, the proximity of antibacterial hand sanitiser to clinic rooms, the location of the sharps disposal container, infection control regarding the movement of cystic fibrosis patients throughout the building, the accessibility of resuscitation bags, and the impact of the building's climate on testing reagents.[60] In a subsequent paper, Colman et al. offer guidelines for simulation-based testing of clinical systems to develop, implement, and evaluate newly built clinical environments using principles and tools derived from the Agency for Healthcare Research and Quality.[40]

An iterative approach to testing and embedding was evident in the response to the COVID-19 pandemic, when many healthcare workflows and practices had to be rapidly adjusted to minimise infection risks.[25,61] Simulation strategies were used to explore the risks of COVID-19 transmission within current practices, and to assess changes designed to reduce risks at the individual, team, and system level. Some initially promising interventions, such as Perspex boxes to protect airway teams from exposure to COVID-19 during intubation, turned out not to be effective or feasible when tested in simulated practice.[50]

Box 5 describes a hypothetical case vignette in which a design thinking approach is used to rapidly design a fever clinic for COVID-19 testing, drawing on anecdotal experience of colleagues during the COVID-19 pandemic.

Simulation can be used proactively to test and refine planned changes in specific contexts, but the generalisability of the findings is not always straightforward. For example, the findings of simulations of the effectiveness of specific cognitive aids in helping to select paediatric anaesthesia equipment in one hospital may, if the human factors principles are the same, be useful across multiple contexts. But the success of modifications to a massive transfusion protocol developed through simulation may depend on the interrelationships of that care pathway with local hospital systems, teams, and capabilities, and hence require development and testing at a local level.

3.4 Helping Healthcare Professionals to Learn about and Embed a Culture of Improvement

Learning about the theory and practice of healthcare improvement is now a requirement in many undergraduate and postgraduate training programmes in medicine and other health professions.[62] Simulation techniques can support experiential methods of education on reporting and investigating patient safety incidents, process mapping, plan-do-study-act cycles, intervention design, and culture change.[63] Simulation-based activities can invite practitioners to reflect on their practice through a quality and safety lens and the actions and behaviours that might be needed to improve it. In one study involving a collaborative ethnography of a trauma service, on-the-ground care providers with no formal role in healthcare improvement reflected that a programme of regular in situ simulation allowed them to feel engaged in 'process review and improvement' and empowered teams to form a habit of 'team reflection'.[20] Other examples involve inviting professionals to explore problems such as emergency room crowding or hospital-acquired infections using tabletop or computer simulations. In these exercises, professionals are asked to develop and undertake healthcare improvement efforts that have consequences as the simulation unfolds. After the simulation exercise, they take part in facilitated reflection on the impacts of their improvement efforts in the example and to draw out wider learning. Another useful technique is debriefing to marginal gains – that is, exploring what went well and what could go just 1% better at an individual, team, or systems level. This is a simple way to inspire an improvement mindset in individuals and teams and further support the cultural foundation of a Safety II approach. The hypothetical case vignette described in Box 6 illustrates how a mindset can be engendered in simulation and then translated to learn from real patient care.

> Box 5 Rapid design of a fever clinic
>
> At the onset of the COVID-19 pandemic, representatives of a hospital, a public health unit, and paramedics in a Canadian city collaborated to design and implement a fever clinic, where community members could attend for COVID-19 testing if they developed concerning symptoms. To meet the rapidly escalating demand for COVID-19 testing, conception to rollout took just 3 days. There were many practical considerations and environmental barriers to ensuring efficient flow and safety of patients in an unconventional space.
>
> The stakeholder team used multiple simulation methods to support a design thinking approach to create the clinic. First, a large venue – an ice hockey arena – was identified as the city location most accessible to the general public. The team brainstormed potential options for flow through the space using a tabletop and to-scale mock-up, taking into account the need to facilitate a one-way flow while maintaining social distancing and minimising contact between providers and patients. This exercise enabled the team to identify three possibilities for the most ideal use of the space.
>
> The next day, the team went to the site to test the three different plans using 20 actors to simulate patients. Stakeholders from each of the groups involved in providing care were present and took part in the exercise. Collectively, they identified that the second option – entrance and exits at opposite ends of the arena, and a two-stage approach to assessment and swabbing – was most efficient and safe. Simulated patients and staff were able to provide further information about what would make the experience better. These considerations were taken into account when the final infrastructure was put in place for opening the next day. During the clinic's first week, members of the team were on site; they interviewed patients and staff and facilitated debriefs at the end of each day. The process and space were adapted in real time in response to user experience.

When simulation is used to explore and enhance healthcare performance in this way, it has the added benefit of *signalling improvement as a priority* and may also contribute to changing the safety culture of the system.[33]

4 Critiques of Simulation

This section offers critiques of published literature and examples through an effectiveness, efficiency, and return-on-investment lens. We explain some

BOX 6 DEBRIEFING TO MARGINAL GAINS

For years, a hospital emergency department has run a weekly simulation programme for registrars (emergency medicine trainees) and nurses with typical resuscitation cases. The simulation facilitators decide to debrief to marginal gains for a period of 6 months after hearing about the theory at a conference. This involves asking the groups to collectively reflect on what could have gone 1% better during the simulated case as part of the regular weekly debrief. They do not plan to measure any specific outcomes.

One evening, a patient with an ST elevation myocardial infarction (STEMI) arrives in the department during a very busy shift. There is a delay in getting the patient to the catheterisation lab. At the end of the shift, the attending physician overhears a casual conversation between one of the emergency nurses and a registrar. The nurse has initiated a conversation with the registrar by saying: 'That was a hard night, what do you think we could have done 1% better for that patient with the STEMI?' Both the nurse and the registrar were able to identify small, individual improvements within their control that could have facilitated more streamlined and timely care. This reflection has become a habit engendered by the simulation.

practical considerations for and barriers to the delivery of simulation as an improvement technique, including cost, faculty development (for simulation delivery teams), technical issues, safety risks, and ethical considerations. We consider the connection between simulation and healthcare improvement – as fields of practice and scholarship, governance relationships within institutions, and a comparison of tools, terminology, and frameworks. We discuss how simulation may influence other organisational learning approaches, such as clinical event debriefing programmes.

4.1 Is Simulation an Effective Technique for Improvement?

The challenges of evaluating simulation as an educational technique have been extensively discussed,[64] and similar challenges surface when considering evaluation of simulation-based interventions for healthcare improvement. Given the variety of techniques encompassed by the term simulation and the diverse contexts in which the method may be applied, no single study is likely to provide the answer to what works and why in simulation, notwithstanding some interesting examples.[26,41,45]

Potential unintended *negative* consequences of simulation in the setting of healthcare improvement remain underreported and underexplored. Simulation can be intuitively appealing as a safe approach to improvement – practising skills and teamwork seem likely to improve performance, and practising on plastic manikins or with actors who simulate patients seems inherently safer than with real patients. But there are also well-described safety risks of conducting simulation activities.[65,66] Ironically, for example, in situ simulation exercises can themselves pose a potential threat to safe and efficient service delivery to real patients in clinical areas: by deploying staff from clinical care into a simulation, by preventing a real patient from using a physical space, and by mixing simulated and real equipment and medications.[65] Simulation programmes have adopted systems and processes to mitigate these risks, including the development of formal no-go criteria for cancelling in situ simulation exercises,[66] and guidance on developing simulation safety policies.[67] If simulation sessions are poorly facilitated, there are also potential threats to the psychological safety of teams, which could have downstream effects on patient safety.

Simulation will always be an imperfect recreation of the complex healthcare environment, and there are risks of embedding bad habits (e.g. medical students not wearing gloves in simulation) or even perpetuating culturally embedded bias or prejudices (e.g. using predominantly white-skinned and male manikins).[68] Growing interest in equity, diversity, and inclusion within healthcare has prompted important reflection among simulation facilitators,[69] and there is increasing interest in simulation as a technique for addressing equity, diversity, and inclusion issues.[70]

One challenge for evaluation is that simulation is often used as one part of a more comprehensive improvement strategy.[45] While often pragmatic and appropriate, it can complicate efforts to evaluate the specific contribution of the simulation elements to the outcomes.[26] As such, it can be difficult to determine the interrelationships between findings from exploratory simulation *informing* other improvement strategies, versus simulation design *being informed* by data collected as part of the broader improvement effort.[17] Even though academic reports commonly separate or seek to separate the two cleanly, the reality is that simulation may have roles in both *informing* and *being informed by* other healthcare improvement efforts that cannot easily be distinguished.[53,54]

4.2 How Should We Integrate Simulation into Healthcare Improvement?

The integration of simulation into the healthcare improvement strategies of organisations offers considerable potential but is often not fully realised.

Aligning simulation with contemporary approaches to healthcare improvement is important, and should prevent conflicting or competing agendas, philosophies, or claims on resources. For example, testing whether planned interventions are feasible, acceptable, or effective in simulated environments and teams aligns well with the Safety II approach to focusing on 'work as done' rather than 'work as imagined'.[18] Barlow et al.[55] use language and tools drawn from healthcare improvement when outlining a framework for documenting and reporting latent system threats unearthed during simulation scenarios. Drawing on human factors and plan-do-study-act constructs, the framework supports the capture and reporting of findings on system deficits to key decision-makers. Connecting simulation-based approaches to other improvement initiatives within an organisation can help in the same way. For example, simulation experts with skills in managing reflective conversations might take a lead in developing clinical event debriefing programmes for healthcare teams, which can be used to discuss opportunities for improvement after real patient care encounters.

However, barriers in integrating simulation-based strategies in overarching healthcare improvement approaches are posed by different traditions of scholarship and practice.[26] This may be manifest in disconnected terminology and in organisational structures and professional groups. With some notable exceptions,[71] healthcare management journals tend not to cover simulation-based healthcare improvement. Within organisations, simulation programmes may be situated in educational structures and staffed by educational experts, while healthcare improvement teams may use tools and language unfamiliar to simulation delivery teams or clinicians. Where a simulation programme sits within a healthcare organisation, it will tend to drive both the organisation's focus and sphere of influence.[72] Simulation programmes that have weaker links to the quality and operational structures within their organisation are less likely to help inform the organisation's strategic direction.

The consumer voice has not been well established in design or delivery of simulation activities, either for education or for improving quality and safety. Drawing on established frameworks for healthcare consumer engagement,[73] there clearly is a role for consumers in simulation design, delivery, and strategy development,[74] but it so far appears to be a missed opportunity.

While the field continues to develop, the questions posed in Box 7 may be helpful. Also important is recognition that skills in running simulations – including design and execution of scenarios, skills in managing debriefing or reflective practice conversations, and systems-focused debriefing[3] – are highly specialised and require specific training. Although simulation techniques are varied and evidence of the relative benefits of various simulation methods to achieve improvement is still emerging, we do know that it is essential for the

> BOX 7 QUESTIONS TO HELP ENSURE GOOD PRACTICE WHEN USING SIMULATION
> AS A HEALTHCARE IMPROVEMENT TECHNIQUE
>
> • Is simulation the right method to address this issue?
> • What are the explicit and specific objectives of the simulation?
> • Are we effectively matching objectives to our simulation technique(s)?
> • Who should be involved in the design, delivery, and debriefing processes?
> • How are we going to measure and understand impact?
> • What are the potential unintended consequences?
> • How does simulation fit into the larger healthcare improvement plan?

goals to be clearly defined and the design to be feasible and cost-effective to implement.[17,28]

4.3 Can We Build a Business Case for Simulation?

While there is increasing awareness of simulation as a quality and safety technique, building a business case for simulation at scale remains challenging. Simulation activity is often resource-intensive, and, for all its potential to improve quality, there are significant downsides to simulation. Activities can be expensive – for example, in relation to equipment, staff time, and use of clinical areas for simulation. There is also limited information about what dose and frequency of simulation is effective. Recruiting and training simulation facilitators to the required level of expertise in both simulation techniques and the skills needed for clinical redesign and healthcare improvement is difficult.

Evidence of return on investment may therefore be much in demand, but little published data are yet available.[75] The lack of evidence arises partly because of the emerging nature of the field and because some important impacts of simulation and debriefing are in areas such as team trust and psychological safety, which are difficult to place on a balance sheet. Lin et al.[76] offer steps to gather the necessary information to conduct an economic evaluation of simulation-based education programmes and curricula, and describe the main approaches to conducting an economic evaluation.

A useful framework is offered by Shah and Course to 'help identify, understand, and evaluate return on investment from large-scale application of [quality improvement]'.[77] It describes six domains:

- patient, carer, and family experience outcomes
- staff experience
- productivity and efficiency
- cost avoidance
- cost reduction
- revenue.

Although the framework has limitations, including the absence of links to patient outcomes and provider effectiveness, it encourages a focus on domains that the clinicians undertaking improvement-focused simulation work may not instinctively think about. We encourage those involved in healthcare improvement simulations to begin framing design and measurement of impact around these domains to support a business case for simulation in their organisation.

In Box 8 we apply the Shah and Course framework to two of our prior hypothetical examples.

BOX 8 APPLYING THE SHAH AND COURSE FRAMEWORK[77] TO HYPOTHETICAL EXAMPLES

Team Training Related to Cardiac Arrest in Patients after Cardiac Surgery (Box 1)

Return on investment could be considered through the primary domains of patient, carer, and family experience outcomes and through staff experience. The simulation programmes should be co-designed by simulation providers and the target units to ensure that the intervention is relevant to their goals as a group. This will maximise staff engagement and ensure that it meets their objectives. Collaborative design and facilitation may demonstrate organisational support and commitment to employees and enhance provider experience. Measuring the impact of the simulation activity could include simple patient metrics (e.g. rate of return of spontaneous circulation and survival after cardiac arrest, time to delivery of epinephrine in anaphylaxis), but also in numerous ways that the staff experience could be measured. The researchers should collaborate with social scientists to apply frameworks such as relational coordination theory,[78] which allows for the quantification of the quality of working relationships between groups, or to conduct interviews and focus groups that explore the relationship between simulation and the psychological safety of the team. The impact of in situ simulation activities on patients and families on the wards where these programmes are run would be a further avenue to demonstrate impact.[79]

Task Trainers to Improve Operating Theatre Efficiency (Box 2)

Return on investment could be considered though the domains of productivity and efficiency, cost reduction, and revenue. This intervention was specifically designed to improve operating room efficiency, but there was no measurable improvement at an organisational level. Anecdotally, engaged residents seemed to perform more efficiently. This negative study provides valuable insight. Not surprisingly, without appropriate, thoughtful, supportive infrastructure (i.e. curriculum and credentialing) the cost of providing LapSim trainers to residents does not outweigh the benefit for the hospital. The next step would be to understand whether more defined, milestone-based curriculum for residents and a credentialing process can translate into organisationally relevant outcomes. In measuring the impact of the simulation activity, those tasked should go beyond operating theatre metrics (e.g. time on the table, cases per day) and collaborate with healthcare finance experts to evaluate the impact on cost reduction (per case) and revenue generated through increased turnover.

The application of return-on-investment frameworks to simulation activity is unfamiliar territory for many of those who plan and facilitate simulation. This highlights why early collaboration between simulation facilitators, those with improvement expertise, and those with skills in economic evaluation should be the standard for simulation programmes seeking to demonstrate return on investment.

5 Conclusions

Simulation offers considerable potential as a technique for improving quality and safety in healthcare. Achieving its full potential will require building on the success of simulation as an educational strategy, and shifting from description of project exemplars towards building consensus on theory and principles to guide practice. It will also require engaging with questions on when and how simulation is the right method to address a particular issue, which design factors might influence success, how effectiveness should be measured, and how to mitigate potential unintended consequences.

Future research should see direct and purposeful collaboration between those with expertise in healthcare improvement and those with expertise in simulation in a deliberate effort to understand, explore, and capitalise on the different theoretical foundations of these fields. Healthcare organisations should make the intersection of these agendas and skills a priority in organisational structures. The potential impacts are more likely to be achieved if simulation-based approaches can demonstrate a multifaceted return on investment and are aligned with other improvement initiatives at institutional and national levels.

6 Further Reading

- Brazil et al.[26] – an overview of the connection between healthcare simulation and healthcare improvement, as fields of practice and scholarship.
- Maxworthy et al.[80] – a comprehensive overview of the field of healthcare simulation practice.
- Brazil[17] – defines translational simulation, and describes a conceptual reframing of how simulation can contribute to healthcare improvement.
- Nickson et al.[30] – an operational framework and practical toolkit for simulation applied to improving quality in healthcare.
- Key professional organisations in the field of healthcare simulation practice:
  - Society for Simulation in Healthcare: www.ssih.org
  - Society for Simulation in Europe: www.sesam-web.org

Contributors

All authors contributed to the design, structure, and writing of each section of the Element, and have approved the final version.

Conflicts of Interest

Victoria Brazil is Medical Director of the Gold Coast Health Simulation Service, Director of the Bond Translational Simulation Collaborative, co-producer of Simulcast, and Senior Editor at *Advances in Simulation*. Eve Purdy is an emergency physician at Gold Coast University Hospital, and a Research Fellow within the Bond Translational Simulation Collaborative. Komal Bajaj is Chief Quality Officer for NYC Health + Hospitals/Jacobi, Clinical Director for the NYC Health + Hospitals Simulation Center, Professor of Obstetrics & Gynecology at Albert Einstein College of Medicine, on the Editorial Board of *Simulation in Healthcare*, and a member of the Board of Trustees for the Center for Medical Simulation.

Acknowledgements

We thank the peer reviewers for their insightful comments and recommendations to improve the Element. A list of peer reviewers is published at www.cambridge.org/IQ-peer-reviewers.

Funding

This Element was funded by THIS Institute (The Healthcare Improvement Studies Institute, www.thisinstitute.cam.ac.uk). THIS Institute is strengthening the evidence base for improving the quality and safety of healthcare. THIS Institute is supported by a grant to the University of Cambridge from the Health Foundation – an independent charity committed to bringing about better health and healthcare for people in the UK.

About the Authors

Victoria Brazil is Professor of Emergency Medicine and Director of the Translational Simulation Collaborative at Bond University, and a senior staff specialist in emergency medicine at Gold Coast University Hospital. Her main interests are connecting education with patient care – through healthcare simulation, team development, and podcasting.

Eve Purdy is an applied anthropologist and Emergency Medicine Consultant at Gold Coast University Hospital. She is interested in understanding how relationships impact teamwork and the role of simulation in team performance.

Komal Bajaj is Chief Quality Officer at NYC Health + Hospitals/Jacobi/NCB, Clinical Director of NYC Health + Hospitals Simulation Center, and Professor of Obstetrics and Gynecology at Albert Einstein College of Medicine. Her research interests include ingraining equity into healthcare quality, building agency, and simulation as an improvement tool.

Creative Commons Licence

References

1. Lioce L (editor), Lopreiator J (founding editor), Downing D, et al. *Healthcare Simulation Dictionary* (2nd ed.). Rockville, MD: Agency for Healthcare Research and Quality; 2020. www.ssih.org/dictionary (accessed 4 December 2020).

2. Gaba DM. The future vision of simulation in health care. *Qual Saf Health Care* 2004; 13(suppl 1): i2–10. https://doi.org/10.1136/qshc.2004.009878.

3. Dubé MM, Reid J, Kaba A, et al. PEARLS for systems integration: a modified PEARLS framework for debriefing systems-focused simulations. *Simul Healthc* 2019; 14: 333–42. https://doi.org/10.1097/sih.00000000000 00381.

4. McGaghie WC, Issenberg SB, Cohen ER, Barsuk JH, Wayne DB. Does simulation-based medical education with deliberate practice yield better results than traditional clinical education? A meta-analytic comparative review of the evidence. *Acad Med* 2011; 86: 706–11. https://doi.org/ 10.1097/ACM.0b013e318217e119.

5. Nestel D, Bearman M, editors. *Simulated Patient Methodology: Theory, Evidence and Practice*. Chichester: John Wiley & Sons; 2014. https://doi. org/10.1002/9781118760673.

6. Zary N, Johnson G, Boberg J, Fors UG. Development, implementation and pilot evaluation of a web-based virtual patient case simulation environment – Web-SP. *BMC Med Educ* 2006; 6: 10. https://doi.org/10.1186/ 1472-6920-6-10.

7. McGaghie WC, Draycott TJ, Dunn WF, Lopez CM, Stefanidis D. Evaluating the impact of simulation on translational patient outcomes. *Simul Healthc* 2011; 6: S42–7. https://doi.org/10.1097/SIH.0b013e318222fde9.

8. Issenberg SB, McGaghie WC, Petrusa ER, Lee Gordon D, Scalese RJ. Features and uses of high-fidelity medical simulations that lead to effective learning: a BEME systematic review. *Med Teach* 2005; 27: 10–28. https:// doi.org/10.1080/01421590500046924.

9. Motola I, Devine LA, Chung HS, Sullivan JE, Issenberg SB. Simulation in healthcare education: a best evidence practical guide. AMEE Guide No. 82. *Med Teach* 2013; 35: e1511–30. https://doi.org/10.3109/0142159x.2013 .818632.

10. Institute of Medicine. *To Err Is Human: Building a Safer Health System*. Washington, DC: The National Academies Press; 2000. https://doi.org/ 10.17226/9728.

11. Lacerenza CN, Marlow SL, Tannenbaum SI, Salas E. Team development interventions: evidence-based approaches for improving teamwork. *Am Psychol* 2018; 73: 517–31. https://doi.org/10.1037/amp0000295.

12. Baker DP, Day R, Salas E. Teamwork as an essential component of high-reliability organizations. *Health Serv Res* 2006; 41: 1576–98. https://doi.org/10.1111/j.1475-6773.2006.00566.x.

13. King HB, Battles J, Baker DP, et al. TeamSTEPPS™: team strategies and tools to enhance performance and patient safety. In: Henriksen K, Battles JB, Keyes MA, Grady ML, editors. *Advances in Patient Safety: New Directions and Alternative Approaches* (Vol 3: Performance and Tools). Rockville, MD: Agency for Healthcare Research and Quality; 2008: 5–20. www.ncbi.nlm.nih.gov/books/NBK43665 (accessed 9 October 2022).

14. Figueroa MI, Sepanski R, Goldberg SP, Shah S. Improving teamwork, confidence, and collaboration among members of a pediatric cardiovascular intensive care unit multidisciplinary team using simulation-based team training. *Pediatr Cardiol* 2013; 34: 612–9. https://doi.org/10.1007/s00246-012-0506-2.

15. Meurling L, Hedman L, Sandahl C, Felländer-Tsai L, Wallin CJ. Systematic simulation-based team training in a Swedish intensive care unit: a diverse response among critical care professions. *BMJ Qual Saf* 2013; 22: 485–94. https://doi.org/10.1136/bmjqs-2012-000994.

16. Reason J. Human error: models and management. *BMJ* 2000; 320: 768–70. https://doi.org/10.1136/bmj.320.7237.768.

17. Brazil V. Translational simulation: not 'where?' but 'why?' A functional view of in situ simulation. *Adv Simul* 2017; 2: 20. https://doi.org/10.1186/s41077-017-0052-3.

18. Hollnagel E, Wears RL, Braithwaite J. *From Safety-I to Safety-II: A White Paper*. www.england.nhs.uk/signuptosafety/wp-content/uploads/sites/16/2015/10/safety-1-safety-2-whte-papr.pdf (accessed 9 October 2022).

19. Wheeler DS, Geis G, Mack EH, LeMaster T, Patterson MD. High-reliability emergency response teams in the hospital: improving quality and safety using in situ simulation training. *BMJ Qual Saf* 2013; 22: 507–14. https://doi.org/10.1136/bmjqs-2012-000931.

20. Brazil V, Purdy E, Alexander C, Matulich J. Improving the relational aspects of trauma care through translational simulation. *Adv Simul* 2019; 4: 10. https://doi.org/10.1186/s41077-019-0100-2.

21. Macrae C, Draycott T. Delivering high reliability in maternity care: in situ simulation as a source of organisational resilience. *Saf Sci* 2019; 117: 490–500. https://doi.org/10.1016/j.ssci.2016.10.019.

22. Dieckmann P, Patterson M, Lahlou S, et al. Variation and adaptation: learning from success in patient safety-oriented simulation training. *Adv Simul* 2017; 2: 21. https://doi.org/10.1186/s41077-017-0054-1.

23. Dubé M, Posner G, Stone K, et al. Building impactful systems-focused simulations: integrating change and project management frameworks into the pre-work phase. *Adv Simul* 2021; 6: 16. https://doi.org/10.1186/s41077-021-00169-x.

24. Auerbach M, Kessler DO, Patterson M. The use of in situ simulation to detect latent safety threats in paediatrics: a cross-sectional survey. *BMJ Simul Technol Enhanc Learn* 2015; 1: 77–82. https://doi.org/10.1136/bmjstel-2015-000037.

25. Brazil V, Lowe B, Ryan L, et al. Translational simulation for rapid transformation of health services, using the example of the COVID-19 pandemic preparation. *Adv Simul* 2020; 5: 9. https://doi.org/10.1186/s41077-020-00127-z.

26. Brazil V, Purdy EI, Bajaj K. Connecting simulation and quality improvement: how can healthcare simulation really improve patient care? *BMJ Qual Saf* 2019; 28: 862–5. https://doi.org/10.1136/bmjqs-2019-009767.

27. Fent G, Blythe J, Farooq O, Purva M. In situ simulation as a tool for patient safety: a systematic review identifying how it is used and its effectiveness. *BMJ Simul Technol Enhanc Learn* 2015; 1: 103–10. https://doi.org/10.1136/bmjstel-2015-000065.

28. Petrosoniak A, Brydges R, Nemoy L, Campbell DM. Adapting form to function: can simulation serve our healthcare system and educational needs? *Adv Simul* 2018; 3: 8. https://doi.org/10.1186/s41077-018-0067-4.

29. Posner GD, Clark ML, Grant VJ. Simulation in the clinical setting: towards a standard lexicon. *Adv Simul* 2017; 2: 15. https://doi.org/10.1186/s41077-017-0050-5.

30. Nickson CP, Petrosoniak A, Barwick S, Brazil V. Translational simulation: from description to action. *Adv Simul* 2021; 6: 1–11. https://doi.org/10.1186/s41077-021-00160-6.

31. Lamé G, Dixon-Woods M. Using clinical simulation to study how to improve quality and safety in healthcare. *BMJ Simul Technol Enhanc Learn* 2020; 6: 87–94. https://doi.org/10.1136/bmjstel-2018-000370.

32. LeBlanc VR, Manser T, Weinger MB, et al. The study of factors affecting human and systems performance in healthcare using simulation. *Simul Healthc* 2011; 6: S24–9. https://doi.org/10.1097/SIH.0b013e318229f5c8.

33. Patterson MD, Geis GL, Falcone RA, LeMaster T, Wears RL. In situ simulation: detection of safety threats and teamwork training in a high

risk emergency department. *BMJ Qual Saf* 2013; 22: 468–77. https://doi.org/10.1136/bmjqs-2012-000942.

34. Purdy EI, McLean D, Alexander C, et al. Doing our work better, together: a relationship-based approach to defining the quality improvement agenda in trauma care. *BMJ Open Qual* 2020; 9: e000749. https://doi.org/10.1136/bmjoq-2019-000749.

35. Lawton R, Taylor N, Clay-Williams R, Braithwaite J. Positive deviance: a different approach to achieving patient safety. *BMJ Qual Saf* 2014; 23: 880–3. https://doi.org/10.1136/bmjqs-2014-003115.

36. Baxter R, Lawton R. The positive deviance approach. In: Dixon-Woods M, Brown K, Marjanovic S, et al., editors. *Elements of Improving Quality and Safety in Healthcare*. Cambridge: Cambridge University Press; 2022. https://doi.org/10.1017/9781009237130.

37. Braithwaite J, Wears RL, Hollnagel E. Resilient health care: turning patient safety on its head. *Int J Qual Health Care* 2015; 27: 418–20. https://doi.org/10.1093/intqhc/mzv063.

38. Sørensen JL, Østergaard D, LeBlanc V, et al. Design of simulation-based medical education and advantages and disadvantages of in situ simulation versus off-site simulation. *BMC Med Educ* 2017; 17: 20. https://doi.org/10.1186/s12909-016-0838-3.

39. Rosen MA, Hunt EA, Pronovost PJ, Federowicz MA, Weaver SJ. In situ simulation in continuing education for the health care professions: a systematic review. *J Contin Educ Health Prof* 2012; 32: 243–54. https://doi.org/10.1002/chp.21152.

40. Colman N, Doughty C, Arnold J, et al. Simulation-based clinical systems testing for healthcare spaces: from intake through implementation. *Adv Simul* 2019; 4: 19. https://doi.org/10.1186/s41077-019-0108-7.

41. Ajmi SC, Advani R, Fjetland L, et al. Reducing door-to-needle times in stroke thrombolysis to 13 min through protocol revision and simulation training: a quality improvement project in a Norwegian stroke centre. *BMJ Qual Saf* 2019; 28: 939–48. https://doi.org/10.1136/bmjqs-2018-009117.

42. Knobel A, Overheu D, Gruessing M, Juergensen I, Struewer J. Regular, in-situ, team-based training in trauma resuscitation with video debriefing enhances confidence and clinical efficiency. *BMC Med Educ* 2018; 18: 127. https://doi.org/10.1186/s12909-018-1243-x.

43. Andreatta P, Saxton E, Thompson M, Annich G. Simulation-based mock codes significantly correlate with improved pediatric patient cardiopulmonary arrest survival rates. *Pediatr Crit Care Med* 2011; 12: 33–8. https://doi.org/10.1097/PCC.0b013e3181e89270.

44. Steinemann S, Berg B, Skinner A, et al. In situ, multidisciplinary, simulation-based teamwork training improves early trauma care. *J Surg Educ* 2011; 68: 472–7. https://doi.org/10.1016/j.jsurg.2011.05.009.

45. Long E, Cincotta DR, Grindlay J, et al. A quality improvement initiative to increase the safety of pediatric emergency airway management. *Paediatr Anaesth* 2017; 27: 1271–7. https://doi.org/10.1111/pan.13275.

46. Griswold-Theodorson S, Ponnuru S, Dong C, et al. Beyond the simulation laboratory: a realist synthesis review of clinical outcomes of simulation-based mastery learning. *Acad Med* 2015; 90: 1553–60. https://doi.org/10.1097/acm.0000000000000938.

47. Goldshtein D, Krensky C, Doshi S, Perelman VS. In situ simulation and its effects on patient outcomes: a systematic review. *BMJ Simul Technol Enhanc Learn* 2020; 6: 3–9. https://doi.org/10.1136/bmjstel-2018-000387.

48. Lamé G, Simmons RK. From behavioural simulation to computer models: how simulation can be used to improve healthcare management and policy. *BMJ Simul Technol Enhanc Learn* 2020; 6: 95–102. https://doi.org/10.1136/bmjstel-2018-000377.

49. Nataraja RM, Oo YM, Kyaw KK, et al. Clinical impact of the introduction of pediatric intussusception air enema reduction technology in a low- to middle-income country using low-cost simulation-based medical education. *Simul Healthc* 2020; 15: 7–13. https://doi.org/10.1097/sih.0000000000000397.

50. Begley JL, Lavery KE, Nickson CP, Brewster DJ. The aerosol box for intubation in coronavirus disease 2019 patients: an in-situ simulation crossover study. *Anaesthesia* 2020; 75: 1014–21. https://doi.org/10.1111/anae.15115.

51. Purdy E, Borchert L, El-Bitar A, et al. Taking simulation out of its "safe container" – exploring the bidirectional impacts of psychological safety and simulation in an emergency department. *Adv Simul* 2022; 7: 5. https://doi.org/10.1186/s41077-022-00201-8.

52. Mannion R. Making culture change happen. In: Dixon-Woods M, Brown K, Marjanovic S, et al., editors. *Elements of Improving Quality and Safety in Healthcare*. Cambridge: Cambridge University Press; 2022. https://doi.org/10.1017/9781009236935.

53. Liberati EG, Tarrant C, Willars J, et al. How to be a very safe maternity unit: an ethnographic study. *Soc Sci Med* 2019; 223: 64–72. https://doi.org/10.1016/j.socscimed.2019.01.035.

54. Abdelrahman A, Murnaghan M. PRactical Obstetric Multi-Professional Training course. *BMJ* 2013; 346: e8561. https://doi.org/10.1136/bmj.e8561.

55. Barlow M, Dickie R, Morse C, Bonney D, Simon R. Documentation framework for healthcare simulation quality improvement activities. *Adv Simul* 2017; 2: 19. https://doi.org/10.1186/s41077-017-0053-2.

56. Kaba A, Barnes S. Commissioning simulations to test new healthcare facilities: a proactive and innovative approach to healthcare system safety. *Adv Simul* 2019; 4: 17. https://doi.org/10.1186/s41077-019-0107-8.

57. Petrosoniak A, Hicks C, Barratt L, et al. Design thinking-informed simulation: an innovative framework to test, evaluate, and modify new clinical infrastructure. *Simul Healthc* 2020; 15: 205–13. https://doi.org/10.1097/sih.0000000000000408.

58. Marshall SD, Sanderson P, McIntosh CA, Kolawole H. The effect of two cognitive aid designs on team functioning during intra-operative anaphylaxis emergencies: a multi-centre simulation study. *Anaesthesia* 2016; 71: 389–404. https://doi.org/10.1111/anae.13332.

59. Spiegelman J, Sheen JJ, Goffman D. Readiness: utilizing bundles and simulation. *Semin Perinatol* 2019; 43: 5–10. https://doi.org/10.1053/j.semperi.2018.11.002.

60. Colman N, Stone K, Arnold J, et al. Prevent safety threats in new construction through integration of simulation and FMEA. *Pediatr Qual Saf* 2019; 4: e189. https://doi.org/10.1097/pq9.0000000000000189.

61. Brydges R, Campbell DM, Beavers L, et al. Lessons learned in preparing for and responding to the early stages of the COVID-19 pandemic: one simulation's program experience adapting to the new normal. *Adv Simul* 2020; 5: 8. https://doi.org/10.1186/s41077-020-00128-y.

62. Wong BM, Ackroyd-Stolarz S, Bukowskyj M, et al. *The CanMEDS 2015 Patient Safety and Quality Improvement Expert Working Group Report.* Ottawa, ON: The Royal College of Physicians and Surgeons of Canada; 2014. www.royalcollege.ca/rcsite/documents/canmeds/patient-safety-ewg-report-e.pdf (accessed 9 October 2022).

63. Worsham C, Swamy L, Gilad A, Abbott J. Quality improvement virtual practicum: the QI simulator. *MedEdPORTAL* 2018; 14: 10670. https://doi.org/10.15766/mep_2374-8265.10670.

64. McGaghie WC, Issenberg SB, Cohen ER, Barsuk JH, Wayne DB. Translational educational research: a necessity for effective health-care improvement. *Chest* 2012; 142: 1097–103. https://doi.org/10.1378/chest.12-0148.

65. Raemer D, Hannenberg A, Mullen A. Simulation safety first: an imperative. *Adv Simul* 2018; 3: 25. https://doi.org/10.1186/s41077-018-0084-3.

66. Bajaj K, Minors A, Walker K, Meguerdichian M, Patterson M. "No-go considerations" for in situ simulation safety. *Simul Healthc* 2018; 13: 221–4. https://doi.org/10.1097/sih.0000000000000301.

67. Brazil V, Scott C, Matulich J, Shanahan B. Developing a simulation safety policy for translational simulation programs in healthcare. *Adv Simul* 2022; 7: 4. https://doi.org/10.1186/s41077-022-00200-9.

68. Conigliaro RL, Peterson KD, Stratton TD. Lack of diversity in simulation technology: an educational limitation? *Simul Healthc* 2020; 15: 112–14. https://doi.org/10.1097/SIH.0000000000000405.

69. Purdy E, Brazil V, Symon B. Equity, diversity, and inclusion in simulation – a reflexive tool for simulation delivery teams. International Clinician Educators Blog: The Royal College of Physicians and Surgeons of Canada; 14 September 2021. https://icenetblog.royalcollege.ca/2021/09/14/equity-diversity-and-inclusion-in-simulation-a-reflexive-tool-for-simulation-delivery-teams (accessed 9 October 2022).

70. Buchanan DT, O'Connor MR. Integrating diversity, equity, and inclusion into a simulation program. *Clin Simul Nurs* 2020; 49: 58–65. https://doi .org/10.1016/j.ecns.2020.05.007.

71. Dench B, Barwick S, Barlow M. It's time for the mandatory use of simulation and human factors in hospital design. *Aust Health Rev* 2020; 44: 547–9. https://doi.org/10.1071/AH19114.

72. Trawber RAH, Sweetman GM, Proctor LR. Improving simulation accessibility in a hospital setting: implementing a simulation consultation service. *Simul Healthc* 2021; 16: 261–7. https://doi.org/10.1097/sih.00000000000 00497.

73. Carman KL, Dardess P, Maurer M, et al. Patient and family engagement: a framework for understanding the elements and developing interventions and policies. *Health Aff (Millwood)* 2013; 32: 223–31. https://doi.org/10.1377/ hlthaff.2012.1133.

74. Barwick S, Brazil V. 4 tips to safely manage healthcare consumer engagement during in situ simulation. International Clinician Educators Blog: The Royal College of Physicians and Surgeons of Canada; 30 June 2020. https:// icenetblog.royalcollege.ca/2020/06/30/4-tips-to-safely-manage-healthcare-consumer-engagement-during-insitu-simulation (accessed 25 April 2022).

75. Nestel D, Brazil V, Hay M. You can't put a value on that … Or can you? Economic evaluation in simulation-based medical education. *Med Educ* 2018; 52: 139–41. https://doi.org/10.1111/medu.13505.

76. Lin Y, Cheng A, Hecker K, Grant V, Currie GR. Implementing economic evaluation in simulation-based medical education: challenges and opportunities. *Med Educ* 2018; 52: 150–60. https://doi.org/10.1111/medu.13411.

77. Shah A, Course S. Building the business case for quality improvement: a framework for evaluating return on investment. *Future Healthc J* 2018; 5: 132–7. https://doi.org/10.7861/futurehosp.5-2-132.

78. Gittell JH, Godfrey M, Thistlethwaite J. Interprofessional collaborative practice and relational coordination: improving healthcare through relationships. *J Interprof Care* 2013; 27: 210–13. https://doi.org/10.3109/13561820.2012.730564.

79. Yates KM, Webster CS, Jowsey T, Weller JM. In situ simulation training in emergency departments: what patients really want to know. *BMJ Simul Technol Enhanc Learn* 2015; 1: 33–9. https://doi.org/10.1136/bmjstel-2014-000004.

80. Maxworthy JC, Epps CA, Okuda Y, Mancini ME, Palaganas J, editors. *Defining Excellence in Simulation Programs* (2nd ed.). North American edition (August 24, 2022): Lippincott Williams & Wilkins; 2022.

Cambridge Elements ≡

Improving Quality and Safety in Healthcare

Editors-in-Chief
Mary Dixon-Woods
THIS Institute (The Healthcare Improvement Studies Institute)

Mary is Director of THIS Institute and is the Health Foundation Professor of Healthcare Improvement Studies in the Department of Public Health and Primary Care at the University of Cambridge. Mary leads a programme of research focused on healthcare improvement, healthcare ethics, and methodological innovation in studying healthcare.

Graham Martin
THIS Institute (The Healthcare Improvement Studies Institute)

Graham is Director of Research at THIS Institute, leading applied research programmes and contributing to the institute's strategy and development. His research interests are in the organisation and delivery of healthcare, and particularly the role of professionals, managers, and patients and the public in efforts at organisational change.

Executive Editor
Katrina Brown
THIS Institute (The Healthcare Improvement Studies Institute)

Katrina is Communications Manager at THIS Institute, providing editorial expertise to maximise the impact of THIS Institute's research findings. She managed the project to produce the series.

Editorial Team
Sonja Marjanovic
RAND Europe

Sonja is Director of RAND Europe's healthcare innovation, industry, and policy research. Her work provides decision-makers with evidence and insights to support innovation and improvement in healthcare systems, and to support the translation of innovation into societal benefits for healthcare services and population health.

Tom Ling
RAND Europe

Tom is Head of Evaluation at RAND Europe and President of the European Evaluation Society, leading evaluations and applied research focused on the key challenges facing health services. His current health portfolio includes evaluations of the innovation landscape, quality improvement, communities of practice, patient flow, and service transformation.

Ellen Perry
THIS Institute (The Healthcare Improvement Studies Institute)

Ellen supported the production of the series during 2020–21.

About the Series
The past decade has seen enormous growth in both activity and research on improvement in healthcare. This series offers a comprehensive and authoritative set of overviews of the different improvement approaches available, exploring the thinking behind them, examining evidence for each approach, and identifying areas of debate.

Cambridge Elements ☰

Improving Quality and Safety in Healthcare

Elements in the Series

Collaboration-Based Approaches
Graham Martin and Mary Dixon-Woods

Co-Producing and Co-Designing
Glenn Robert, Louise Locock, Oli Williams, Jocelyn Cornwell, Sara Donetto, and Joanna Goodrich

The Positive Deviance Approach
Ruth Baxter and Rebecca Lawton

Implementation Science
Paul Wilson and Roman Kislov

Making Culture Change Happen
Russell Mannion

Operational Research Approaches
Martin Utley, Sonya Crowe, and Christina Pagel

Reducing Overuse
Caroline Cupit, Carolyn Tarrant, and Natalie Armstrong

Simulation as an Improvement Technique
Victoria Brazil, Eve Purdy, and Komal Bajaj

Workplace Conditions
Jill Maben, Jane Ball, and Amy C. Edmondson

Printed in the United States
by Baker & Taylor Publisher Services

Printed in the United States
by Baker & Taylor Publisher Services